I0844035

Nutrition and Fitness on a Budget

High-impact Strategies for Every Wallet

Table of Contents

Chapter 1. Introduction

Welcome to our Special Report on "Nutrition and Fitness on a Budget: High-impact Strategies for Every Wallet"! This is your invaluable guide to achieving and maintaining optimum physical wellness without breaking your bank. No, it's not a highly technical topic, so you need not worry about intricate jargon! It is indeed an exciting, insightful, and thoroughly accessible treasure chest of practical tips, intelligent strategies, and creative solutions. This report is curated for everyone with an urge for a healthier lifestyle, even while sticking to a budget. So, are you ready to embark on this journey towards achieving your health objectives without straining your wallet? Let's redefine the narrative that fitness and nutrition are pricey hobbies—invest in this Special Report, and you'll see the glow of health and wealth radiate in equal measures!

Chapter 2. Understanding Nutrition: The Key to Fitness

Nutrition is the cornerstone of our health. It is the fuel that powers our body's functions, supports our physical performance, and influences our emotional well-being. However, nutrition can often be a complex subject shrouded in misconceptions. To achieve optimum fitness on a budget, it's vital we start with a clear understanding of the basics.

2.1. Fundamentals of Nutrition

Simply put, nutrition refers to the foods we consume, their nutrients, how those nutrients nourish our bodies, and the role these have in our health. The nutrients we receive from our diet are divided into macro- and micronutrients.

Macronutrients are the nutrients we need in large quantities, namely: carbohydrates, proteins, and fats. These are the primary sources of energy that our bodies use to perform various functions.

Micronutrients, though needed in smaller quantities, are essential in supporting our overall health. They include vitamins and minerals and play critical roles in disease prevention, growth, and good health.

2.2. Importance of Balanced Nutrition

The key to maximizing nutrition and fitness is balanced eating. A balanced diet is one that gives your body all the nutrients it needs from a variety of foods in the right proportions.

1. **Carbohydrates**: Typically, about half of your calories each day should come from carbohydrates. They are vital for energy production and brain function.

2. **Protein**: Provides the building blocks for body tissues and is also used for energy. Men and women aged 19–50 should consume about 46–56 grams of protein per day, respectively.

3. **Fats**: Essential for many body processes, including hormone production. Fats should make up about a third of your daily intake.

4. **Fibers**: Naturally found in foods such as fruits, vegetables, and whole grains. They are essential for healthy digestion.

5. **Vitamins and Minerals**: They play numerous roles in the body, from maintaining bone health to boosting the immune system.

Balanced nutrition is about more than just counting calories. The quality of your calorie intake matters – opting for nutrient-dense foods can offer more health benefits than foods high in empty calories. Understanding this concept is one of the key strategies to eating well on a budget.

2.3. Nutrition and Physical Performance

Nutrition plays a pivotal role in our physical performance, influencing energy levels, endurance, muscle strength, and recovery.

Protein, for instance, is crucial for building and repairing tissues, particularly muscle tissue. Having sufficient protein before and after workouts supports muscle recovery and growth.

Carbohydrates are your body's go-to fuel during high-intensity workouts. Ensuring enough carbohydrate intake can mean the difference between ending a workout energetically or hitting an energy wall.

Remember, inadequate or poor dietary intake can lead to nutrient deficiencies, limiting your physical performance and, over time, potentially leading to more serious health problems.

2.4. Eating Healthy on a Budget

The common misconception is that eating healthy is expensive, but cost-effective nutritional strategies can help you stay on a budget while maximizing nutritional intake. Here are some tips:

1. **Plan Meals**: Plan meals around whole, nutrient-dense foods that are in season or on sale.

2. **Bulk Buying**: Buy in bulk, but ensure these are items that won't spoil readily, such as grains, pasta, or canned goods.

3. **Cook At Home**: Control costs and know what's in your food by cooking more at home.

4. **Utilize Frozen or Canned Produce**: These are often just as nutritious as fresh produce but often come at a fraction of the price.

2.5. Supplements: Do You Need Them?

Supplements can be a controversial topic. They are popular among athletes and fitness enthusiasts but shouldn't replace balanced nutrition.

Supplements can be handy in specific situations, like iron supplements for those with anemia or protein supplements for athletes who struggle to meet their protein needs through food. However, indiscriminate use of supplements can lead to adverse effects and undermine food-first approaches to nutrition.

Always consider your dietary needs, lifestyle, and budget before deciding to take supplements. Never underestimate the power of a balanced diet, adequate rest, and regular exercise in achieving optimal health.

In conclusion, understanding nutrition and its interplay with fitness is fundamental to achieving and maintaining good health. A balanced diet can be the key to optimal performance and recovery, while strategic grocery shopping and meal planning can make healthy, nutrient-dense diets achievable even on a tight budget. Investing the time to understand, practice, and balance the principles of good nutrition won't only contribute to your physical well-being but to your financial health as well.

Chapter 3. Breaking Down the Myth: Fitness ≠ Expensive

The notion that a fit and healthy lifestyle is expensive is pervasive and commonly unchallenged. Exotic "superfoods", high-end gym memberships, and premium wellness programs can put you back hundreds, if not thousands, of dollars. But achieving and maintaining optimum health doesn't have to burn a hole in your pocket. Let's debunk this myth together, showing how smart strategies, a pinch of creativity, and a dash of self-discipline can help keep your body and bank in top shape!

3.1. Unearthing the Roots of the Myth

The axiom 'Fitness is Expensive' was not born overnight. It's a perception we've crafted over decades, fueled by advertising, mainstream media, and an overall emphasis on the "premium" aspect of health and wellness. Marketers sell us fancy gym-equipments, diet plans, and workout apparel that we "absolutely need" to stay fit. The reality, however, is that while these luxuries can aid in fitness, they're not necessary or defining factors for a healthy lifestyle.

3.2. Smart Shopping = Nutritious and Affordable Eating

Smart and sensible shopping is the key to unlock a treasure chest of nutritious and affordable food.

- Seasonal and Local Produce: Vegetables and fruits that are in season and locally grown are generally more affordable than those flown halfway around the globe. Plus, they're fresher, packing in more essential nutrients.

- Bulk Buying: Opt for bulk buying for staples like rice, pasta, beans, and lentils. Buying in large quantities usually means a lower cost per unit, savings that quickly add up over time.

- Cook at Home: Not only is home cooking considerably cheaper than eating out, but it also lets you control your ingredient quality and quantity.

3.3. Budget Fitness: No Gym, No Problem!

Who said you need an expensive gym membership to stay fit? Physical fitness can be achieved through numerous free or inexpensive means.

- Bodyweight Exercises: Push-ups, planks, squats, and lunges are examples of exercises that use your body weight for resistance and can be done anywhere.

- Outdoor Activities: Running, biking, swimming in public pools, hiking trails, or even brisk walking are excellent ways to stay fit.

- Online Resources: Numerous free online resources offer workout tutorials, fitness videos, and yoga classes. These online platforms make fitness affordable and accessible to all.

3.4. Investing in Durable Workout Wear and Gear

While it's tempting to splurge on the latest fitness fad, your wallet will thank you if you invest in high-quality, durable workout wear and gear that will last longer.

- Buy Essentials First: Start with the basics like a good pair of sports shoes, a few moisture-wicking clothes, and a reusable water bottle. As you develop your fitness routine, invest in additional equipment or attire as needed.

- Opt for Durable Brands: Instead of going for the most trending brands, select quality brands known for their durability and long-lasting performance.

3.5. Demystifying the "Health Food" Hype

You don't need to invest in exotic "superfoods" or expensive protein powders for a healthy diet. Yes, these can nourish you, but there are numerous affordable alternatives that are equally nourishing.

- Simple is Often Better: Fresh fruits, vegetables, whole grains, and lean proteins are the foundation of a healthy diet. These are usually more affordable and just as nutritious as trendy health foods.

- DIY Protein Shakes: You can make your protein shakes at home using ingredients like peanut butter, greek yogurt, and milk, instead of expensive commercial protein powders.

3.6. The Power of Planning and Discipline

One of the most impactful strategies that wouldn't cost a cent is being organized and disciplined.

- Plan Your Meals: Planning your meals for the week can help you avoid the cost and unhealthy trap of takeaways and processed foods.

- Regular Exercise Routine: Consistency is more critical than intensity when it comes to exercise. A regular home-based or outdoor workout routine is all you need to remain fit.

By transforming these strategies from words to actions, dispelling the myth, "Fitness ≠ Expensive" would be effortless. In the journey of fitness on a shoe-string budget, remember, the ultimate secret lies not in the contents of your wallet, but in the resolve of your mind!

By redefining norms and reimagining what fitness and wellness mean, we move closer to a world where health is inclusive, affordable, and achievable for everyone. And in this world, wallets don't become thinner while waistlines get trimmer! Your health and wealth are a pair, and they can grow hand in hand.

Chapter 4. Strategizing Your Meals: Eating Healthy on a Shoestring

Eating healthy on a shoestring budget can seem challenging, but these strategies can help you achieve your health goals while staying financially smart.

4.1. Start With a Plan

Before hitting your local grocery store, take the time to create a detailed meal plan. Knowing what you're going to cook and eat not only helps you maintain a healthy diet but also prevents overspending. Determine what meals and snacks you'll be having for every day of the week and list down all the ingredients you need. Consider your schedule too. If you know you don't have time to cook from scratch every day, factor in some easy, fast meals like salads using leftovers or budget-friendly slow-cooker recipes.

Building a balanced meal plan on a budget means incorporating various affordable nutritious foods. Consider these categories:

- Lean Proteins: Eggs, tofu, lentils, or beans.
- Whole Grains: Brown rice, oats, whole grain pasta, or quinoa.
- Fresh Vegetables and Fruits: Opt for locally grown ones as they're usually cheaper.
- Healthy Fats: Avocado, olive oil, nuts, and seeds.

4.2. Shop Smart

Once your meal plan is in place, the next step is savvy shopping. Be cost-conscious without compromising healthy options. Here are a few strategies:

1. Use coupons and discounts: Always check for coupons, discounts, and sales in your local grocery stores. But remember, only buy discounted items that are already a part of your meal plan.

2. Buy in bulk: Getting non-perishable items like grains, pasta, or canned beans in bulk is cheaper over time than buying smaller amounts.

3. Choose seasonal produce: Fruits and vegetables that are in season generally cost less and are more nutritionally rich.

4. Buy whole foods: Precut fruits, vegetables, or grains may save you prep time, but cost significantly more.

5. Go meatless: Regularly swapping out meat for plant-based proteins like lentils or chickpeas can substantially reduce your grocery bill.

4.3. Cooking at Home and Meal Prep

Learning to cook at home can offer significant savings over pre-made meals and dining out. Start small by learning a few recipes that you enjoy and gradually expand your repertoire.

Investing a few hours in meal prep over the weekend can help you save both time and money during the week. Prepare multiple portions of a meal at once and store them in the fridge or freezer for later use. This way, you have a healthy, home-cooked meal ready when you're pressed for time.

4.4. Leftovers Are Your Friend

One of the easiest ways to make your meals more cost-effective is to plan for leftovers. This could mean intentionally cooking extra, or using yesterday's leftovers to make today's meal. Making one pot dishes such as stew, chili, or rice dishes often leaves you numerous servings for a reduced cost.

4.5. Healthy Eating Out

Yes, it's possible to eat out healthily and cost-effectively. If you must eat out, look for restaurants that support your health and budget goals. Take advantage of lunch specials, share dishes, or divide your meal in half for another meal. Opt for water instead of expensive beverages and avoid superfluous extras like appetizers and desserts.

4.6. Growing Your Own Food

Starting a small vegetable and herb garden can be a fulfilling and cost-effective way to encourage healthy eating. Nothing promotes health and well-being more than eating homegrown produce. Even if you don't have a lot of space, consider container gardening or growing herbs on your windowsill.

Remember, eating healthy on a budget is a journey of many steps. Don't expect to perfect all these strategies overnight. Start with implementing a few and gradually incorporate more as they become second nature.

Eating healthily doesn't need to be an expensive proposition. With careful planning, smart shopping, and a bit of creativity, you can enjoy a variety of nutritious meals without burning a hole in your wallet. It's about making smart, conscious decisions that will foster a healthy body, a peaceful mind, and a well-managed budget—and this guide offers steps to help you achieve just that.

Chapter 5. Smart Shopping: How to Buy What You Need without Overspending

A smart shopper can fill the kitchen with nutritious foods and aids without spending exorbitantly. This involves strategic planning, knowing your needs, and understanding the value of foods and items for fitness. The following guide will show you, step-by-step, how to achieve this efficiently and effectively.

5.1. Understand the Nutritional Values

First things first, it's essential to understand the nutritional value of different types of foods. This knowledge arms you with the information you need to make smart choices when shopping. For instance, brown rice and quinoa may be more expensive than white rice, but they offer more nutritional benefits such as higher fiber content, proteins, and lower glycemic index. Therefore, it means you're getting more value for your money, not just a lower price, making them a wiser purchase.

5.1.1. The Nutritional Values of Healthy Foods

Here are some typical healthy choices and their nutritional values:

- Quinoa: Rich in fiber, magnesium, B-vitamins, iron, potassium, calcium, phosphorus, vitamin E and antioxidants.

- Lentils: Good source of protein, fiber, iron, and potassium.

- Lean meats: High in protein, vitamin B, iron, potassium, and zinc.

- Fruits: Full of essential vitamins and minerals, fiber,

antioxidants, and low in calories.

- Vegetables: Abundant in vitamins, minerals, fiber, and antioxidants, while also being low in calories.

Prioritizing these types of foods gives you more nutritional bang for your buck.

5.2. Learn to Plan and Prepare

Meal planning and preparation not only save you money by preventing waste but also ensure you always have healthy, nutritious meals on hand. You will be less tempted to buy expensive pre-made meals or order takeout.

5.2.1. Basic Steps in Meal Planning and Preparation

Here is a step-by-step guide to efficient meal planning:

1. Write down the meals you want to cook for the week.
2. List all necessary ingredients.
3. Check your pantry, fridge, and freezer to see what you already have.
4. Update the list to only include what needs to get purchased.
5. Stick to this list when you go shopping.

This plan prevents impulse purchases, saving you money, and ensuring ingredients get fully used before they spoil.

5.3. Time Your Purchases Right

Making purchases at the right time can significantly cut your spending. For example, buying fruits and vegetables in their peak season or during a sale can save you money and offer optimal flavor and nutrition.

5.3.1. Seasonal Buying Guide

Here's a basic guide outlining when certain fruits and vegetables are in season:

Spring: * Fruits: Apricots, cherries, strawberries. * Vegetables: Asparagus, peas, lettuce, new potatoes.

Summer: * Fruits: Blackberries, blueberries, melons, peaches, raspberries. * Vegetables: Aubergine, bell peppers, courgettes, tomatoes.

Autumn: * Fruits: Apples, cranberries, pears, plums. * Vegetables: Butternut squash, mushrooms, pumpkin, sweetcorn.

Winter: * Fruits: Clementines, grapefruit, kiwi. * Vegetables: Brussels sprouts, cauliflower, leeks, winter squash.

5.4. Capitalize on Sales and Discounts

Sales are a great way of saving money. Store loyalty cards, bulk purchase discounts, and other in-store promotions can lower overall costs. However, ensure these sales apply to nutritious foods – buying unhealthy discounted foods will not contribute to your health goals.

5.5. Invest in Fitness Equipment Wisely

When it comes to fitness equipment, understanding your needs and researching different options are crucial. Choose equipment that matches your fitness level and goals, and look for good quality second-hand items or sales to save money.

In conclusion, smart shopping involves understanding nutritional values, planning and preparing meals, timing purchases correctly, taking advantage of sales and discounts, and making wise investments in fitness equipment. By applying these principles, it's possible to maintain your fitness and nutrition goals without overspending.

Chapter 6. Meal Prepping: Your Wallet's Best Friend

The concept of meal prepping is becoming progressively popular in the realm of nutrition and fitness. No longer exclusive to fitness aficionados or weight-loss champions, it's being embraced by a diverse range of individuals. Why? Because it enables achieving a healthier lifestyle in a cost-effective way.

This treasure trove of a concept can keep you on track with your dietary goals, save you time, and most importantly, reduce your food costs significantly. Let's delve deeper into understanding the art and science of meal prepping and how it can become your wallet's best friend.

6.1. Understanding Meal Prepping

Meal prepping simply means planning and preparing your meals in advance. It usually involves determining the week's menu, shopping for the ingredients, and then cooking and storing the food. You can prep for every meal of the day, including snacks, or just focus on the ones that you struggle with. For many, that's often lunch.

Meal prepping is not about crafting gourmet meals for each day. Instead, it's about creating simple, nutritious, and tasty food that can be easily reheated and consumed. The key concept here is forward-thinking, which can save you immense stress, time, and money.

6.2. Why Meal Prepping is Cost-Effective

When we buy food in bulk, we often get it at a reduced cost. By planning your meals ahead, you can intelligently utilize these bulk purchases throughout your meals, swiftly cutting your per meal cost.

Apart from this, meal prepping curtails impulsive food ordering or unhealthy snacking, both of which can quickly add up costs. Lastly, if food is ready and waiting, there's a smaller chance you'll let it spoil. This reduces food wastage, another check for your wallet!

6.3. Getting Started with Meal Prepping

Your meal prepping journey starts with understanding your dietary needs and identifying the meals you want to prep. Are you targeting weight loss? Or perhaps, aiming for muscle gain? Or maybe you just want to maintain a balanced diet. Different goals require different nutrition plans.

6.4. Step 1: Plan Your Meals

A good start is to pick one or two days in a week for meal prepping. Sunday and Wednesday are common choices, depending upon your schedule.

You may start with planning for a couple of days and gradually extend it to cover the entire week. Use a meal chart, a simple grid on paper or an app on your phone, whatever you feel comfortable with, to schedule your meals.

Choose recipes that you like and keep your nutritional goals in mind. Include a balance of proteins, carbs, and fats, and remember to add variety to your menu to keep it interesting and wholesome.

6.5. Step 2: Make your Shopping List

Once you have your meal plan, the next step is drafting your shopping list. Categorize the list by the grocery store sections, like produce, dairy, grains, meats, and snacks. This will prevent any last-minute rushed additions.

Remember to check your pantry before you head to the store, to avoid buying ingredients you already have.

6.6. Step 3: Smart Shopping

One of the significant advantages of meal prepping is that you can make efficient use of bulk purchases. Buy larger quantities of staple items like rice, pasta, lentils, or anything you use frequently.

Pay attention to the per unit cost highlighted on the price tag. Just because something is in bulk doesn't necessarily mean it's cheaper.

Try to aim for versatile ingredients. For example, chicken can be used in a salad, a sandwich, or a mainland dish. Such ingredients can create a variety of dishes without burning a hole in your pocket.

6.7. Step 4: Cook and Store

Once you've got all your ingredients together, it's time to start cooking. Simplify the process by categorizing the tasks. Begin with washing and cutting all the produce, then start cooking, perhaps beginning with the items that take the longest to cook. In the end, pack and store the meals in appropriate containers.

Remember that some foods, like salads or fruits, are better fresh. Store ingredients for such meals individually, and combine them only at mealtime.

6.8. Meal Prepping Tips for More Savings

Now that we've mastered the basics, let's discuss some savvy tips to extract maximum value from your meal prepping routine.

1. Stick to In-Season Produce: In-season fruits and vegetables are fresher, tastier, and cheaper. An additional benefit is that they change through the year, providing a natural variation to your diet.

2. Go Vegetarian at Times: Meat is usually the most expensive component of a meal. Including a few vegetarian meals in your week can help lower the cost.

3. Freeze: If you find a great deal, buy in bulk and freeze. Freezing preserves most foods without reducing their nutritional value.

4. Grow Your Own: If possible, grow your own herbs and vegetables. It's always cheaper, and the fresh taste is unbeatable!

5. Leftovers as Ingredients: Be creative and use your dinner leftovers for an exciting lunch the next day. This can add a fun twist to your meals and save money!

To conclude, meal prepping is a versatile and highly beneficial strategy that can lower your food costs while improving your nutrition and health. Integrating it into your routine might seem daunting at first, but with a bit of practice, it can become a fun and vital part of your wellness journey.

Chapter 7. Effective Home Workouts: No Gym Membership Needed

Keeping healthy and fit doesn't have to mean an expensive gym membership. There are plenty of cost-effective ways to exercise at home, often using items you already have. Let's explore these strategies for staying healthy and fit, no gym membership needed.

7.1. The Power of Bodyweight Exercises

Bodyweight exercises are an excellent place to start for home fitness. These types of workouts don't require any equipment, are highly versatile, and accommodate all fitness levels.

Some popular bodyweight exercises you can do at home include: push-ups, planks, squats, and lunges. These exercises primarily target the chest, abdominal muscles, legs, and glutes, but they also engage other muscle groups, helping you achieve a full-body workout without ever stepping foot in the gym.

There's a variety of ways to adjust these exercises according to your fitness level. For instance, if you're a beginner, you can start with wall push-ups rather than traditional push-ups. Similarly, you can begin with planks performed on your knees.

7.2. Build Your Own Circuit Training

Circuit training is highly effective as it combines cardiovascular exercise with strength training. This form of exercise will help you burn calories and build muscle without any specialized equipment.

The ideal way to create a circuit is to choose five or more exercises that you can perform without breaks lasting 30 seconds to a minute. After completing each exercise, take a break for a minute or two, then start another circuit. Repeat the entire circuit three to four times.

Here's an example of a circuit you might assemble:

1. 30 seconds of jumping jacks

2. 30 seconds of push-ups

3. One minute of plank

4. 30 seconds of squats

5. 30 seconds of lunges

6. One minute of rest

Repeat the above circuit three to four times.

Circuit training allows you to tweak the sequence according to your preferences or switch out exercises as needed, providing flexibility and versatility.

7.3. Harness The Power of HIIT

High-Intensity Interval Training (HIIT) is a time-efficient workout method that alternates between intense bouts of exercise and short recovery periods. It is particularly effective for improving cardiovascular health and boosting metabolism.

A simple HIIT sequence might look like this:

1. 30 seconds of sprinting (in place, if necessary)

2. Minute of slow walking or rest

3. Repeat for 15-20 minutes

HIIT sessions are typically shorter compared to other workout sessions, so they're an excellent option for those who are short on time.

7.4. Make the Most of Household Items

You don't need to shop for expensive weights or machines. The items around your house can serve as excellent makeshift workout equipment.

For example, a solid chair can be used to do tricep dips and step-ups. Cans of food, bottles of water, or bags of rice can act as weights for performing bicep curls or shoulder press exercises. Even a pair of socks on a tiled or hardwood floor can help you perform an intense core-sliding workout.

7.5. Take Advantage of Online Resources

You do not need personal trainers when you have an abundance of resources available at your fingertips—most of them free. Online platforms such as YouTube are brimming with guided workout videos for various fitness levels and styles. You can find everything from five-minute ab workouts to one-hour full-body yoga sessions.

Remember, being on a budget shouldn't impede your fitness journey. With a little creativity and determination, you can build a high-impact, effective workout routine right at home, without stepping into a gym or draining your wallet. Stay active, stay healthy!

Chapter 8. Make Your Calorie Count: Cost-Effective Nutritious Foods

Eating healthily doesn't mean you have to splurge on expensive food items. Even with a limited budget, you can effectively nourish your body with just the right nutrients. The key is to make your calories count, to choose foods with high nutritional value per dollar by considering their nutrient density. This approach ensures that you get more bang for your buck, thus maximizing every calorie consumed.

8.1. Picking Nutrient-Dense Foods

Nutrient-dense foods are those that deliver high proportions of essential nutrients in relation to their calorie content. In other words, they contain more vitamins, minerals, dietary fiber, and other essential nutrients for fewer calories. To capitalize on these supple sources of nutrients without splurging, here are some great whole foods that you should incorporate into your diet.

1. **Legumes**: Beans, lentils, and peas are excellent sources of plant-based proteins and fiber which are perfect for a budget-conscious diet. They are also packed with complex carbohydrates to keep you satiated for a long time. This, in turn, can help to control food quantity and manage weight.

2. **Eggs**: These are a staple that should never be underestimated. Easily accessible and rich in high-quality protein, choline, selenium, and various B vitamins, eggs are affordable and extremely versatile — ideal for varied meals every time!

3. **Whole Grains**: Brown rice, oats, barley, and quinoa are not only more nutritious but are also more filling than the refined options.

They are excellent sources of fiber, B vitamins, and several minerals, such as zinc, iron, magnesium, and selenium.

4. **Fruits and Vegetables**: Regardless of your budget, there will always be a set of fruits and vegetables you can afford. Not only are they packed with essential vitamins and minerals, they also contain dietary fiber that aids digestion and makes you feel full, thus preventing overeating.

8.2. Stretch Your Budget by Planning and Purchasing Wisely

Knowing which foods give the most nutrients per dollar is only half of the battle. It's equally important to plan your meals and purchase wisely.

1. **Buy in Bulk**: Identify the staple foods in your diet and try to buy them in large amounts. This approach often provides savings and ensures a consistent supply of these foods.

2. **Purchase Seasonal Produce**: Buying fruits and vegetables that are in season can help you save money since abundant supply often means lower prices. Additionally, these items are often at their peak in terms of nutritional value.

3. **Prepare Your Meals at Home**: Preparing your meals at home allows for significant savings and control over food portions and ingredients. By cooking larger quantities, you can save leftovers for following meals or freeze them for future use.

8.3. Smart Substitutions for High-Cost Items

Incorporating cheaper alternatives to pricier foods in your diet could mean significant savings for your wallet.

1. **Swap Meat for Plant-Based Proteins**: Substituting meat with plant-based proteins such as beans, lentils, or tofu occasionally can reduce expenditure. These can be filling and nutritious options, with the added benefit of being low in saturated fats.

2. **Substitute Fresh Fruits with Frozen or Canned Ones**: If fresh fruits are pricey, consider frozen or canned fruits that retain most of the nutritional benefits. However, ensure that those products do not contain added sugars or high levels of sodium.

8.4. Impact of Cooking Methods on Nutrient Retention

The way you prepare food can influence its nutritional content. Therefore, it's important to employ techniques that enhance or retain the nutrients.

1. **Steam or Blanch Vegetables**: These methods help retain the nutritional value of vegetables while reducing the need for added fats.

2. **Grill, Broil or Roast Meats**: Such methods lower the fat content in the meat by allowing excess fat to drip away.

3. **Use Cooking Liquids**: Save the water used to boil or steam foods, as it can contain vitamins that were released from the food during cooking. You can utilize this nutrient-rich liquid in broths, soups, or sauces.

While healthy eating and nutritious food may seem synonymous with high costs, there's a wealth of choice available for those who are resourceful enough to look and creative enough to capitalize. The tips and practices shared in this section should not only help you make your calories count but also make significant strides in leading an active, productive, and wholesome life, all within a wallet-friendly budget!

Chapter 9. Deciphering Food Labels: Finding Hidden Gems in the Supermarket

Starting your journey to fitness and nutrition does not mean you have to spend hordes of money on organic or exotic foods. One key to making economical and healthy food choices is understanding food labels.

9.1. Understanding the Nutrition Facts Label

The nutrition facts label is an excellent tool to assess the nutritional content of food and beverages. It usually comprises of:

1. Serving Size: Shows the average amount a person would eat. Comparisons among different products should be made using similar serving sizes.

2. Calories: Reflects the number of calories in each serving. The general guide is that 40 calories per serving is considered low, 100 calories is moderate, and 400 or more is high.

3. Nutrients: Describes the number of certain nutrients, e.g. fats, sodium, and fiber, per serving. The values are often in grams, but sometimes as percentages. Having a grasp of these can shape your overall dietary plan.

9.2. Dietary Guidelines

Certain parts of the label have special relevance to dietary planning:

1. % Daily Value: The '% Daily Value' shows how much a nutrient in

a serving of food contributes to a total daily diet. A 5% Daily Value of a nutrient per serving is considered low, while 20% or more is high.

2. Less: Opt for foods low in saturated fat, trans fat, cholesterol, and sodium.

3. More: Aim for foods high in dietary fiber, vitamins, and minerals.

9.3. Unveiling Marketing Tactics

It's common for food companies to use marketing tactics by highlighting specific nutritional benefits. This may not reflect the full nutritional profile of the product. To save money and ensure a healthy purchase, decipher these phrases:

1. "Low Fat" or "Fat-Free": These products can still be high in sugar and calories.

2. "Made with Real Fruits": This does not mean the product is high in fiber. Check the label for dietary fiber content.

3. "Natural": The term "natural" can be misleading as there are no strict regulations for its use.

9.4. A Quick Guide to Food Additives

Food additives are substances added to maintain or improve safety, freshness, taste, texture, or appearance. Some commonly used additives are:

1. Preservatives: Help prevent food spoilage.

2. Sweeteners: Add sweetness with or without the extra calories.

3. Color Additives: Used for visual appeal.

4. Flavors and Spices: Enhance taste.

5. Flavor Enhancers: Enhance the flavors of foods.

6. Texture Agents: Provide desired texture.

Always check for food allergies and intolerances when reading about additives.

9.5. Health Claims

Health claims are often placed in larger or bolder text on packaging. Two types are 'authorized health claims' that are backed by scientific consensus and 'qualified health claims' requiring more research. Be aware of this differentiation when considering product value.

9.6. Staying Vigilant Against Allergens

For individuals with food allergies, reading food labels plays a vital role. Major food allergens, such as wheat, shellfish, peanuts, and eggs, must be listed in simple terms either in the ingredient list or after the list.

9.7. Understanding Ingredients List

The ingredients of a product are listed by weight in descending order. So, those listed first make up a large proportion of the product. Watch out for unhealthy ingredients listed within the top three.

9.8. A Closer Look at Sugars

It's important to differentiate between naturally occurring sugars and added sugars. Fruits contain natural sugars, while soft drinks commonly contain added sugars. 'Total sugars' on a label includes both types.

Eating healthier and staying fit does not demand a colossal budget. With an understanding of food labels, you are well-equipped to make frugal yet nutritious choices in the supermarket. By applying these strategies, you are one step closer to achieving optimum wellness without breaking your bank.

Chapter 10. Balancing Time and Money: Quality Fitness in Less Time

Time is money, and many of us feel like we don't have enough of either. While it's true that you can't create more hours in the day, you can learn to use the time you have more efficiently. The following tips and strategies will help you maximize your time, and get the most benefit from your fitness efforts.

10.1. Budget and Time Friendly Exercises

To best utilize your time and money, choose exercises that provide the maximum benefit for the least amount of time and money spent. Here are a few exercises that are both time and budget-friendly:

1. Running: All you need is a good pair of running shoes and some open space. Running improves cardiovascular health, helps to alleviate stress, burns calories, and doesn't require expensive equipment or gym memberships.

2. Bodyweight exercises: Push-ups, sit-ups, lunges, squats, and similar exercises don't require any equipment. Use your body weight to build strength, improve flexibility, and burn fat.

3. High Intensity Interval Training (HIIT): This involves short bursts of high-intensity exercise followed by short recovery periods. HIIT can be adapted to many types of exercise, is efficient, burns a lot of calories, and yields significant fitness gains.

10.2. Making the Most of Short Workout Times

Many people feel that they don't have time to exercise, but there are plenty of ways to fit fitness into a busy schedule. Here's how to do it:

1. Prioritize workouts: Treat workouts as an unmovable part of your schedule. Make a commitment to yourself and prioritize your health.

2. Utilize breaks: Use coffee breaks, lunch breaks, or any short downtime for quick workouts. A few minutes of activity can add up over time.

3. Work out at home: Save travel time by exercising at home. There's no shortage of free online workouts that cater to various fitness levels and preferences.

4. Multitask: Listen to educational podcasts or audio books, watch the news, or do professional reading while you exercise.

10.3. Investing in Quality, Not Quantity

Don't feel that you need to spend hours in the gym to be fit. Instead, focus on the quality of your workouts. High-intensity, targeted workouts can give better results than lengthy, unfocused workouts. This approach can lead to better progress, reduce risk of injury, and save you both time and money in the long run.

10.4. Making Economical Choices

Fitness doesn't have to be expensive. With a little creativity and resourcefulness, you can maintain a fitness routine on a budget. Here are some tips:

1. Opt for free or inexpensive workouts: As already mentioned, many fitness activities require little to no equipment. Make use of free online resources for workout guides and routine ideas.

2. Buy equipment second-hand or on sale: If you do decide to purchase equipment, look for second-hand items or sales to save money.

3. Share a personal trainer or join a class: Sharing the cost of a personal trainer with a friend or joining a group class can make fitness more affordable.

10.5. Practical Tips for Eating Healthy on a Budget

Nutrition plays a crucial role in fitness. Here are some tips for eating healthy without emptying your wallet:

1. Plan meals: Weekly meal planning reduces impulse purchasing and food waste, and ensures you have the ingredients for healthy meals on hand.

2. Buy in bulk: Foods such as rice, beans, lentils, and oats are often cheaper in bulk. These foods are also nutritious and versatile.

3. Opt for seasonal and local produce: These are generally cheaper and fresher than out of season produce.

4. Prepare your own meals: Eating out is expensive and often less healthy. Cooking at home is good for both your wallet and your waistline.

In conclusion, time and money should not serve as hindrances to achieving fitness. With smart strategies, it's possible to stay on track and achieve your health goals without straining your budget. Always remember that investing in your health is one of the best decisions you'll ever make.

Chapter 11. Maintaining the Momentum: Sustaining Fitness and Nutrition on a Budget

Every healthy lifestyle journey begins with a crucial step—the decision to commit to wellness. But how does one continue this commitment without breaking the bank nor succumbing to boredom or frustration? Don't worry; we have your back with this comprehensive guide on sustaining fitness and nutrition on a budget.

11.1. The Art of Meal Planning

Meal planning is key in maintaining nutrition while keeping an eye on the budget. This simple strategy prevents impulse purchases and ensures you're eating healthy, cost-effective meals throughout the week. At the heart of meal planning are a few pivotal steps:

1. Start by assessing what you already have. Make a list of items in your pantry, fridge, and freezer.

2. Next, decide on a variety of meals for the coming week. Consider how to incorporate the ingredients you already have. Remember, variety isn't just the spice of life, but it ensures varied nutrients too.

3. Draft your shopping list, considering your meal plan and sticking staunchly to it at the store.

11.2. Shopping Habits That Save

Smart grocery shopping plays a significant role in sticking to your budget and ensuring nutritious eating. Here are some habits you should cultivate:

1. Buy in bulk. Bulk shopping saves money and reduces packaging waste.

2. Opt for generic brands. They offer the same nutritional value as pricier name-brand products.

3. Choose seasonal produce. They're cheaper, taste better,and have the highest nutritional value.

4. Don't fear the freezer. Frozen fruits and vegetables are usually just as nutritious as the fresh stuff, and they're reasonably priced.

11.3. Home Cooking: A Healthy and Affordable Choice

Cooking at home provides control over ingredients, portion sizes and costs. Experiment with diverse healthy recipes - the internet is a treasure trove of them. Prepare large quantities and save leftovers for future meals.

11.4. Fitness for Less

Fitness doesn't necessarily mean expensive gym memberships. There are many affordable or free alternatives to stay fit:

1. Outdoor workouts — running, cycling, or hiking.

2. Bodyweight exercises — push-ups, squats, and planks.

3. Online workout videos.

4. Community fitness classes, including yoga and aerobics.

11.5. Keep Moving

Stay active throughout the day. Convert mundane activities into fitness opportunities. Walk or cycle to work, use stairs instead of elevators, do chair exercises while watching TV.

11.6. Repurpose, Recycle, and Reuse in Fitness

Consider repurposing everyday items in your workout regime. A filled water bottle can become a dumbbell, a chair can help with step-ups and tricep dips, stairs can substitute a cardio machine.

11.7. Nurturing Your Mind

Mental wellness plays a significant role in maintaining physical health and fitness momentum. Mindfulness, meditation, and adequate sleep are vital.

11.8. Celebrate Every Victory

Every step towards a healthy lifestyle, no matter how small, warrants celebration. It fuels motivation and more importantly, recognizing your own effort is great for mental wellness.

11.9. Community Effect

Joining fitness and nutrition communities, whether online or offline, can boost your motivation. They can offer support, trade tips, and foster accountability.

11.10. Setting and Pursuing Goals

Set achievable goals, tracking them over time. Evaluate and readjust these goals periodically to align with your changing lifestyle and fitness level.

11.11. Inculcating the Habit of Regular Medical Check-ups

To ensure that your budget-friendly health and fitness practices are positively impacting your health, make sure to incorporate regular medical check-ups into your routine. These can be essential in catching any potential health problems early and addressing them effectively.

Remember, a healthy lifestyle doesn't have to be expensive. Your commitment and a bit of creative thinking can lead to incredible health benefits while not straining your wallet. You've got this!

www.ingramcontent.com/pod-product-compliance
Lightning Source LLC
Chambersburg PA
CBHW060859260726
48661CB00008B/3348